HEARING AIDS

HEARING AIDS
Recent
Developments

Arlene C. Neuman

YORK
PRESS

Baltimore • Toronto • Sydney

This book was manufactured in the United States of America. Typography by Brushwood Graphics, Inc., Baltimore, Maryland. Printing by Wilmer Printing, Inc., Timonium, Maryland. Cover design by Joseph Dieter, Jr. Book design by Studio 1812.

ISBN 0-912752-34-3

INTRODUCTION TO THE SERIES MINI MONOGRAPHS IN COMMUNICATION SCIENCES

The field of Communication Sciences, as with many other fields, is being altered dramatically by advances in modern technology. Consider, for example, recent developments in hearing aid technology. Just a few years ago hearing aids consisted of only a few basic components; specifically, a microphone, amplifier, filter, transducer, earmold, and battery. Today hearing aids embody compression amplifiers of various kinds, adaptive filters, noise reducing circuits, a range of different earmold types, and new forms of wireless signal transmission. In addition, digital methods of signal processing are being used increasingly in modern hearing aids. Digitally controlled programmable hearing aids are now commonplace and all-digital hearing aids embodying advanced signal processing techniques for combating feedback and reducing background noise have recently been developed for clinical use.

New methods of audiological measurement, such as the use of otoacoustic emissions for hearing screening, have been developed recently. There is also a growing trend toward computerization and the integration of seemingly different functions in a single instrument, such as combining auditory measurement, hearing-aid prescription and more efficient methods of audiological record keeping in a single system.

Similar advances are taking place in speech and language pathology. In addition to the many devices that have been developed for augmentative communication, sophisticated computer-based systems have been developed recently for speech and language training. Recent advances in computer analysis of language indicate a greater future role for computers in developing more effective procedures for language intervention.

In order to make effective use of these many advances, it is necessary for clinicians to know how to use this new technology. It is particularly important to understand the capabilities of modern technology in a clinical setting, to distinguish between what can and cannot be expected of modern instruments and to know how to make effective use of what is possible.

The purpose of these mini-monographs is to explain recent technological advances in the communication sciences, their underlying concepts and clinical relevance in easy to understand non-technical language. In so doing it is hoped that clinicians and researchers who acquaint themselves with the contents of these monographs will not only develop improved clinical skills in applying this technology, but will also gain a broader and more enduring view of a rapidly changing professional landscape.

Harry Levitt

PREFACE

This is an exciting time for those of us who work with hearing aids. Technological advances have resulted in the development of hearing aids that allow much more flexibility and the possibility of more successful hearing aid fittings for people with diverse types of hearing loss. In the past five years alone, new options are available to the dispenser, which include programmable hearing aids, multimemory hearing aids, and signal-processing hearing aids.

What are these hearing aids? Do they differ from the hearing aids available ten or twenty years ago? How should one prescribe these hearing aids? These are the questions facing dispensers today. The purpose of this monograph is to provide the basis for answering some of these questions by reviewing recent developments in hearing aids and hearing aid measurement techniques.

Preparation of this monograph was supported in part by Grant No. H133E80019 from the National Institute on Disability and Rehabilitation Research.

HEARING AID DESIGN—THE PROBLEMS

Although many hearing-impaired people derive benefit from using an appropriately prescribed hearing aid, there are still many who have difficulty using one. The reason for the lack of success in using a hearing aid may be attributed to several factors: limitations imposed by the auditory system of the listener; limitations imposed by the environmental degradation of the signal before amplification; and limitations imposed by the hearing aid.

The population of potential hearing aid users has both changed and expanded over the years. These changes are due to advances in medicine and in hearing aid technology. For example, years ago many hearing aid users were persons with conductive hearing loss (Davis et al. 1947). Advances in medicine have improved the effectiveness of treatment for many conditions affecting the conductive mechanism. Therefore, few people with purely conductive type hearing loss are now candidates for amplification. Most hearing aid users have sensorineural-type hearing loss. A smaller number of hearing aid users have a mixed-type hearing loss.

The life expectancy of the population in the United States has increased dramatically. The percentage of the population over age 65 has increased from 9% in 1960 to 12.5% in 1990 (United States Bureau of the Census 1990). Members of this older population may exhibit presbycusis, a sloping sensorineural hearing loss typical of aging. Research indicates that subjects with presbycusis form a special subgroup among subjects with sensorineural hearing loss (Bergman 1971; Bergman et al. 1976).

The improvements in amplification systems have also increased the pool of potential hearing aid users. Because early hearing aids offered limited gain and power, only people with mild and moderate degrees of hearing loss found them helpful. With the introduction of better amplifiers and transducers, hearing-impaired persons with severe and profound degrees of loss can be fitted. In addition, people with steeply sloping hearing loss and purely high frequency hearing loss can also be fitted as a result of the filtering technology now used in hearing aids.

1

The fact that the majority of hearing aid users have a sensorineural-type hearing loss and that the hearing loss may vary widely both in degree and configuration complicates matters for the hearing aid designer. Although the label "sensorineural hearing loss" seems to imply a homogeneous subclass of hearing loss, in fact there are large individual differences with reference to the ability of these hearing-impaired persons to understand a speech signal, even if they are matched for degree of hearing loss and configuration. The transmission of sound may be distorted in the ear with sensorineural hearing loss. The nature of the distortion(s) that may occur in the ear with a sensorineural hearing loss has not been clearly identified. Many different types of distortion have been considered including poor frequency selectivity (e.g., Tyler, Fernandes, and Wood 1980), poor temporal resolution (e.g., Tyler and Summerfield 1980), nonlinearities (e.g., Leshowitz and Lindstrom 1977), and broader critical bands (Florentine et al. 1980; Pick, Evans, and Wilson 1977), among others.

One aspect of sensorineural hearing loss that has a direct effect on the comfort of amplification is the reduced dynamic range often associated with this type of loss. In sensorineural hearing loss, the threshold of hearing is elevated, but the tolerance for loud sounds is not usually shifted upward to compensate for the elevated threshold. In fact, in certain persons with sensorineural hearing loss, loudness discomfort levels are obtained at the same or even lower levels than for people without hearing loss. As the degree of hearing loss increases, the dynamic range (the range between the threshold of audibility and the loudness discomfort level) decreases. This reduction of the range of residual hearing poses a special problem for the design and selection of appropriate amplification, because sounds must be amplified in order to be heard, yet inappropriate amplification will make the sound uncomfortably loud.

A common problem faced by hearing aid users is difficulty in using a hearing aid in noisy situations. Listening to speech in a group situation (e.g., a cocktail party) and listening to speech in noise (environmental) have most frequently been identified as major sources of difficulty in adjusting to using a hearing aid in a survey of hearing aid users (Berger et al. 1982). Experimental results substantiate the disproportionate effect of noise on the speech discrimination abilities of persons with sensorineural hearing loss (Carhart and Tillman 1970; Dirks, Morgan, and Dubno 1982; Dubno, Dirks, and Morgan 1984; Keith and Talis 1972; Leshowitz 1977; Plomp 1978). Unfortunately, a certain amount of noise is present in many listening situations faced daily. For example, Pearsons, Bennett, and Fidell (1976) found that the signal-to-noise ratio of conversation in public places averages 5 to 10 dB. According to studies by Tillman, Carhart, and Olsen (1970) and by Gengel

(1971) signal-to-noise ratios on the order of 10 to 15 dB are necessary for the hearing-impaired person listening through a hearing aid.

Reverberation is another type of distortion present in the listener's environment. A temporal form of distortion caused by reflected energy, reverberation prolongs and modifies a signal within an enclosure. While reverberation does not present significant problems to the non-impaired listener in most daily environments, hearing-impaired listeners seem to be particularly susceptible to its effects (e.g., Finitzo-Hieber and Tillman 1978; Nabelek and Mason 1981; Nabelek and Pickett 1974a,b). Furthermore, there is some evidence that characteristics of particular hearing aids may interact with the speech signal already degraded by reverberation effects (Nabelek and Pickett 1974b; Nabelek, Koike, and Wood 1982).

Hearing aids can introduce distortion into the signal. This is of particular concern in the newer hearing aids that implement nonlinear forms of amplification. One result of syllabic compression, for example, is the smoothing of the waveform envelope and of the spectrum. When multiband syllabic compression is used, more of the temporal and spectral information are removed. Plomp has recommended that only slow acting compression be used for this reason (Plomp 1988). Certainly the results of research on multiband compression with many bands support Plomp's contention. The data from experiments with multiband compression with two or three bands do not seem to show degradation as a result of syllabic compression. The issue of interactions between the distortion of the amplified signal and the characteristics of the listener is a subject of research (e.g., Hecox 1988).

Acoustic feedback is a particular problem for hearing aid users with severe and profound degrees of hearing loss. These individuals need substantial amounts of amplification in order to hear. Sound leaking from the earmold may be picked up at the microphone and be re-amplified. In order to minimize the problem of acoustic feedback, these users often must reduce the volume on the hearing aid. This, of course, reduces the amount of gain and may prevent the user from hearing adequately. New solutions to the problem of acoustic feedback have been implemented in recent hearing aids.

RECENT DEVELOPMENTS IN HEARING AIDS

Probably the most obvious change in hearing aids over the last number of years is miniaturization. Body-worn hearing aids are rarely recommended today; but were state-of-the-art only 30 years ago. The body aid was the most commonly used hearing aid style until the 1960s, but is the least commonly used style today. In 1992, a little over 80% of the hearing aids dispensed were in-the-ear (Cranmer-Briskey 1992a).

Years ago, conventional wisdom was that bigger was better. But, along with the reduction in hearing aid size, there has been an improvement in quality. Hearing aids today have wider bandwidths and smoother frequency responses than did the body aids of years ago. These properties are a direct result of the smaller size of the microphones and receivers (Killion 1993). Since the 1970s, the transducers used in hearing aids have been capable of providing a bandwidth of up to 16kHz. This has not translated into hearing aids of similar bandwidths due to the constraints of getting sufficient output at higher frequencies (above 4kHz) and of acoustic feedback. However, the bandwidths of current hearing aids are wider than were available up until 1970 when hearing aids only provided usable gain up to 3000 Hz *by design*.

Another important development has been in the augmentation of the processing done in modern hearing aids. In contrast to older conventional hearing aids that contained a single linear frequency-gain response with output limiting obtained by peak clipping, current hearing aids contain many other capabilities. For example, hearing aids may include multiple memories/programs (e.g., Widin and Mangold 1988), level-dependent changes in frequency response (e.g., Sigelman and Preves 1987; Killion 1990), single or multiband compression (e.g., Laurence, Moore, and Glasberg 1983; Waldhauer and Villchur 1988) noise suppression (e.g., Graupe, Grosspietsch, and Basseas 1987) feedback suppression (e.g., Bisgaard and Dyrlund 1991), and compression limiting.

Modern hearing aids may be categorized as conventional hearing aids or digital hearing aids. Conventional hearing aids utilize analog technology only. As illustrated in figure 1, the conventional hearing aid contains several components: a microphone, an amplifier, a filter, a limiter, and a receiver (a miniature loudspeaker). An acoustic signal reaching the microphone of the hearing aid will be converted to an electrical signal representing the waveform of the signal as a function of time. This electrical signal is amplified, filtered, and then converted back to an acoustic signal.

Digital hearing aids may be categorized further as digitally controlled analog hearing aids (also known as digital/analog hybrid) and digital signal processing hearing aids (also known as all-digital). As can be seen in figure 2 (a and b), digital hearing aids utilize both analog and digital technology. The microphone, amplifier, limiter, and receiver are common to conventional and digital hearing aids. In the digitally controlled analog hearing aid, analog components of the hearing aid such as the amplifier, filter, and the limiter are controlled by a com-

4

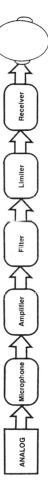

Figure 1. Typical signal path for conventional analog hearing aids. (Reprinted with permission from Hecox and Punch 1988.)

5

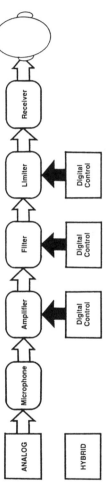

Figure 2a. Typical signal path for digitally controlled analog (digital/analog hybrid) hearing aids. (Reprinted with permission from Hecox and Punch 1988.)

6

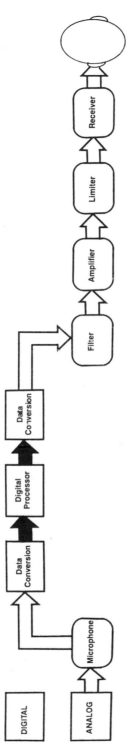

Figure 2b. Typical signal path for digital signal processing hearing aids. (Reprinted with permission from Hecox and Punch 1988.)

puter. The audio signal remains an electric signal and the processing of the signal is done by analog circuitry, but the hardware is controlled by digital circuitry.

Programmable hearing aids are the most commonly found example of the digitally controlled analog hearing aid. In this case, programmable analog filters allow greater flexibility in filtering than does conventional analog circuitry. The digital memory holds the settings for a particular hearing aid. These settings may be changed by reprogramming the hearing aid.

In the hearing aid in which a single set of parameters is stored, the operation of the hearing aid is similar to that of a conventional analog hearing aid. Multimemory, programmable hearing aids provide the option of storing more than one "hearing aid" in memory. The suggestion has been made that these multimemory hearing aids be set up in order to optimize performance in different listening environments. This is analogous to the provision of bifocal eyeglasses, but in the case of hearing aids up to eight memories (possible hearing aids) are available. As yet, studies are not available to provide guidance about how to select the different frequency responses to be included in the hearing aid. Various hearing aid companies have suggested approaches for the fitting of their hearing aids, but evidence for the efficacy of these procedures is lacking.

Programmable hearing aids require a programming unit. Many of the programmable hearing aids can be programmed by the dispenser, rather than the manufacturer. Four different types of programming systems are available: handheld, desktop, PC-based, and remote-controlled (Bisgaard, Christiansen, and Morrison 1993). In some of these systems, a cable connects the programming unit to the hearing aid. The hearing aid is connected to the unit while being programmed and is then disconnected once the programming has been completed. In other systems, the instructions are sent from the programmer to the hearing aid via radio wave or infrared signal.

Programmable systems may be classified further as dedicated systems or multibrand systems. Recently, two different multibrand programming systems have become available. A consortium of several major hearing aid manufacturers developed the PMC (Programmable Multichannel System) (Branderbit 1991). The PMC is a desktop system. Siemens, Rexton, GN Danavox, Phonak, and Philips hearing aids currently have hearing aids programmable with this system (*Hearing Instruments* 1992). The Programmable Fitting System (Swenson) is a PC-based system that can be used with any hearing aid that contains the programmable circuits produced by Intrason France or the Gennum Corporation (Amerine 1992).

Another application of digital technology in the digitally controlled analog hearing aid is the use of digital logic to change the type of filtering that is done in the hearing aid as a function of the incoming signal. This allows more sophisticated types of processing than could be implemented with compression amplification alone. The Zeta Noise Blocker chip introduced in hearing aids in 1986 (Graupe, Grosspietsch, and Taylor 1986) is an example of this type of technology. The Zeta Noise Blocker contains overlapping filters that are controlled by digital circuitry. Digital logic is used to determine whether the sound impinging on the hearing aid within certain bands are signal or noise. If noise is present, that portion of the signal is attenuated.

In the digitally controlled analog hearing aid, the signal remains an analog signal (continuous time-waveform signal). As shown in figure 2b, in the digital signal processing hearing aid, the acoustic signal reaching the microphone is converted to an electrical signal and then is converted to a digital signal—a series of binary numbers. The series of numbers is then manipulated according to a set of instructions known as a signal-processing algorithm. The all-digital hearing aid, thus, contains software in addition to the hardware. The software contains the instructions for manipulating the string of numbers. A digital hearing aid may implement the same types of processing that are currently contained in conventional hearing aids, but also has the potential for much more sophisticated types of processing such as complex forms of noise reduction, speech feature enhancement, and speech recognition and resynthesis (see Williamson and Punch 1990, for a review of such processing).

STYLES OF CONVENTIONAL HEARING AIDS

There are two major hearing aid styles in use today: the in-the-ear and the behind-the-ear aid. Use of in-the-ear aids has been steadily increasing over the past several years. In 1992, in-the-ear hearing aids made up approximately 81.9% of sales (Cranmer-Briskey 1992a). The in-the-ear style has several advantages and disadvantages. An important advantage of this type of hearing aid is that the microphone is placed in the external ear, thus preserving some (or with in-the-canal aids, all) localization cues. The small size of the hearing aid and the fact that it fits inside the external ear make this type of hearing aid cosmetically appealing.

In-the-ear hearing aids have become increasingly powerful with improvements in design. Whereas the early in-the-ear hearing aids provided limited gain and were suitable only for those with mild-to-moderate hearing loss, the present generation of in-the-ear aids can be

9

used by people with more severe degrees of hearing loss. At present, in-the-ear hearing aids are not well suited for persons with profound hearing loss because of their need for substantial amplification. The amount of amplification that can be provided by an in-the-ear aid is limited by the problem of acoustic feedback (reamplification of sound that has leaked from the hearing aid). The small receivers used in today's hearing aids produce a lot of mechanical vibration. This may make the entire hearing aid case vibrate. According to Killion (1993), this vibration is the major cause of acoustic feedback in in-the-ear aids. Acoustic feedback is more likely to occur in an in-the-ear hearing aid than in other style aids because the microphone and receiver are very close to each other in the hearing aid case.

In-the-ear aids have smaller batteries and volume controls than are found on other styles of hearing aids. This may limit the use of this type of hearing aid by persons with limited manual dexterity. Recently, several hearing aid companies introduced remote control units that allow the user to control the volume and/or other controls on the hearing aid. The use of a remote control unit may make operation of in-the-ear aids simpler for this population.

Behind-the-ear hearing aids are suitable for persons with any degree of hearing loss. Until recently the behind-the-ear style was the most commonly used hearing aid. In 1980, behind-the-ear models made up approximately 58% of the hearing aid market (Skafte 1988). By 1992, behind-the-ear aids made up only 16.2% of the market (Cranmer-Briskey 1992a). As the use of the in-the-ear style has increased, the use of the behind-the-ear style has decreased.

There are other styles of hearing aids available (e.g., body aids, eyeglass aids). These other hearing aids, in combination, comprise 1.9% of the market (Cranmer-Briskey 1992a). In the body aid, the microphone, hearing aid circuitry, and batteries are contained in a small box worn at chest level, either in a pocket or in a special harness. A cord connects the box to a button-type hearing aid receiver, which in turn is coupled to an earmold.

Body aids are used primarily by persons with a profound hearing loss, although they might also be used by persons with lesser degrees of hearing loss in cases where it is important to have large user controls and batteries. One advantage of a body aid for persons with profound hearing loss is the increased separation between the microphone and receiver in this type of hearing aid. The microphone is located on the hearing aid case, which is worn at chest level, and the receiver is at ear level. The separation of microphone and receiver allows more amplification before the onset of unstable acoustic feedback. Although the location of the microphone at chest level is advantageous with regard to the reduction of acoustic feedback, this location is not optimal for providing the localization cues that would be available were the micro-phone located on the head.

The eyeglass hearing aid is really a variation of the behind-the-ear aid. The hearing aid is built into the temple of the eyeglass frame. The style is sometimes used for a special type of hearing aid fitting used in cases of unaidable unilateral hearing loss. For the CROS (contralateral routing of signals) fitting, the microphone is placed on the side of the unaidable ear and the signal is sent to the opposite ear. The wiring necessary to route the signal to the contralateral side is contained in the eyeglass frame. Wireless CROS fittings that use FM transmission are used for those who do not wear eyeglasses.

STYLES OF DIGITAL HEARING AIDS

Digital hearing aids have been available since the late 1980s. Digital simulations of hearing aids for research purposes had been in use since the 1970s (e.g., Graupe and Causey 1975; Levitt 1982; Levitt et al. 1986). Experimental wearable units were developed in the early 1980s (e.g., Engebretson, Morely, and O'Connell 1986; Engebretson, Morley, and Popelka 1987; Cummins and Hecox 1987; Nunley et al. 1983). The first commercially available digital hearing aid, the Nicolet Phoenix, was sold for a short time beginning in 1988. The first digitally controlled analog hearing aids became available at about the same time.

The Nicolet digital hearing aid was available only as a body style aid. A behind-the-ear case containing the microphone, receiver, and volume control was connected by a cord to a bodyworn digital pro-cessor. This two-part configuration of the digital hearing aid was due to the fact that the digital portion of the hearing aid and the power supply had not yet been miniaturized sufficiently to fit into a behind-the-ear or in-the-ear case. The Nicolet Phoenix provided flexibility in implementation of the frequency-gain response and contained a proprietary digital noise reduction algorithm. An adaptive paired-comparison fitting procedure was included as part of the program-ming system to assist in the selection of the hearing aid.

A major reason for the lack of success of the all-digital hearing aid in 1988 was the use of a body-worn configuration that many hearing aid users found to be cosmetically unacceptable. At that time, it was not possible to produce a smaller digital hearing aid. The heart of the digi-tal hearing aid is a digital signal processing chip. In 1988, the digital chips being used were rather large and required more current than did analog hearing aid components. The lithium batteries used to power the digital chips were larger than the batteries ordinarily found in hear-ing aids. Since then, digital chips that require less power have been developed. Although these hearing aids still require more current than other hearing aids, it is possible to design digital hearing aids that will fit into a behind-the-ear case.

Currently there is one digital signal processing hearing aid on the market that implements a digital feedback suppression process. The behind-the-ear hearing aid contains an analog-to-digital convertor, a digital-to-analog converter, a test signal generator, a mechanism to estimate the feedback and a digital filter that adapts in order to cancel the feedback (Bisgaard and Dyrlund 1991). This feedback suppression is implemented in a high-power hearing aid and is meant to allow the provision of substantial gain in the high frequencies without acoustic feedback. Field studies with the actual instrument are not yet available.

Digitally controlled analog hearing aids are currently available in behind-the-ear and in-the-ear styles. A recent review in a hearing aid trade journal listed sixteen companies offering hearing aids of both styles. These hearing aids offer options such as multichannel compression, multiple programs, and noise suppression options.

PROCESSING IN HEARING AIDS

Filtering

In the simplest type of hearing aid, a sound is amplified and filtered. The acoustic signal reaching the hearing aid is converted to an electrical signal by the hearing aid microphone. This small signal is then converted into a much larger signal that is sufficient to drive the hearing aid receiver. Usually more energy will be provided at higher frequencies (1000 Hz to 6000 Hz) than at lower frequencies (below 1000 Hz). This differential amplification as a function of frequency is achieved by filtering inside the hearing aid. The amount of amplification and type of filtering provided for a particular hearing aid user will depend on the characteristics of the hearing loss for that individual.

The purpose of filtering is to make sounds audible at all frequencies that are important for speech intelligibility. Because the configuration and degree of hearing loss differ among hearing-impaired people, it is important to have a large number of filter shapes and flexibility in fitting the shape of the filter in a hearing aid. Conventional hearing aids are designed with filters appropriate for hearing-impaired persons with the most common configurations of hearing loss. Filters appropriate for people with flat and mildly sloping hearing loss (i.e., hearing that is better in the low frequencies and poorer in the higher frequencies) are readily available. It is also possible to provide appropriate amplification for those with normal hearing in the low frequencies and a steeply sloping high-frequency hearing loss. Recently, solutions to the problem of fitting hearing-impaired persons with upward sloping hearing loss (i.e., hearing that is poorer in the low frequencies and better in the higher frequencies) have been proposed (Killion, Berlin, and Hood 1984). If it is necessary, modifications to the frequency response of the hearing aid may be obtained by use of acoustic dampers and/or manipulation of earmold acoustics.

The new digitally controlled analog hearing aids and digital signal processing hearing aids should make it even simpler to obtain the filter configuration that is optimal for the hearing-impaired user. In cases of unusual audiometric configuration, it may be difficult to obtain an appropriate frequency response with conventional hearing aids. Digital systems have fewer constraints on the filters that can be achieved and should make it possible to provide appropriate amplification in cases of unusual audiometric configuration.

The bandwidth of the hearing aid is also an important consideration. Low-frequency amplification has been shown to be important to the listener's perception of sound quality (e.g., Punch and Beck 1980) and may also contribute to speech intelligibility (e.g., Punch and Beck 1986; Tecca and Goldstein 1984). Mid- and high-frequency amplification have been shown to be important to the listener's speech recognition performance (e.g., Skinner 1980; Skinner, Karstaedt, and Miller 1982; Skinner and Miller 1983).

Until the 1970s, hearing aids had rather narrow bandwidths. With the development of the electret microphone and broadband receivers, hearing aids with bandwidths of up to 20000 Hz are possible (Killion 1982). It is possible to obtain usable amplification at high frequencies when these microphones are used in conjunction with the appropriate earmold configuration (e.g., Killion 1981).

There are practical limitations in implementing broadband hearing aids with large amounts of gain at high frequencies. When large amounts of gain are needed in the high frequencies, two types of problems result: distortion and acoustic feedback. The problem of distortion has most recently been addressed by the development of the class D amplified receiver (Killion 1993).

Provision of usable high-frequency amplification for those with steeply sloping, high-frequency hearing loss is most problematic. Few studies have investigated the specific contribution of the high frequencies (above 2000 Hz) to speech recognition performance. This issue is important because of the great difficulty in obtaining sufficient gain at high frequencies without acoustic feedback. In addition, hearing aid users may object to the quality of amplified speech containing high-frequency emphasis (e.g., the "tinniness" of the hearing aid). Schwartz et al. (1979) compared hearing aids that differed in gain above 2000 Hz.

Better speech recognition performance was obtained with the hearing aid with more high-frequency gain in the noise condition, but not in quiet. Most of the subjects also found the extended high-frequency aid to be of better quality.

Sullivan et al. (1992) used a digital master hearing aid to simulate hearing aids with three different upper cutoff frequencies: 710 Hz, 1790 Hz, and 6000 Hz. Subjects had steeply sloping, high-frequency sensorineural hearing loss. Nonsense syllable recognition was assessed in quiet and in noise at three gain settings. In addition, quality ratings were obtained for both test conditions. Nonsense syllable recognition improved with increasing frequency response, particularly in noise. However, quality ratings decreased when the bandwidth of the hearing aid increased beyond 2000 Hz.

New techniques for feedback suppression have been the subject of much recent research. Both electronic and digital solutions have been proposed. Electronic solutions include notch filter, phase shift, and frequency shift techniques (Preves 1988). Several of the digital solutions have incorporated adaptive filtering techniques. In fact, a digital feedback suppression technique of the adaptive type has now been implemented in a commercially available hearing aid.

Fitting Speech into the Dynamic Range. The signal reaching the hearing aid has substantial variations in level. In the linear hearing aid, the same amount of gain is applied to small signals as is applied to larger signals. This causes problems for some hearing aid users who may need a substantial amount of amplification in order to hear soft sounds, but very little amplification in order to listen to louder sounds. Compression amplification may be used to amplify the signal by differing amounts as a function of the level of the input signal.

Compression is a nonlinear form of amplification. The amount of amplification varies as a function of the input signal. As the input level increases, the amount of gain decreases. The dynamic range of the output signal is, thus, less than that of the input signal. In a compression hearing aid, there will typically be a range of input signals for which the hearing aid will function in a linear mode (i.e., for each increase in input level there will be a fixed increment in output level) and a certain range of input levels for which the hearing aid will operate non-linearly.

Figure 3 illustrates the input-output characteristics of a compression system. Input levels appear on the X-axis and output levels on the Y-axis. For input levels below the *compression threshold,* amplification is linear. For each 10 dB change in input level there is a 10 dB change in output. The compression threshold is the point where compression begins and is defined as that input level at which the gain is 2 dB less than that in the linear region. Above the compression threshold, amplifica-

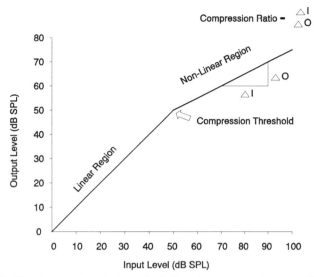

Figure 3. The input-output characteristics of a compression amplifier.

tion is nonlinear. The *compression ratio* is the ratio of the change in input level to the change in output level. In this example, the compression ratio is 2:1. Above the compression threshold, for every 10 dB change in input level, there is a 5 dB change in output.

Compression systems have two time constants: the *attack time* and the *release time*. Attack time is the time delay in initiating the compression. Release time is the time delay in releasing the compression. The method for measurement of attack and release time is specified in ANSI Standard S3.22-1987.

Within the hearing aid, the compression circuit may be placed before the volume control of the hearing aid or after the volume control. The former placement is referred to as *input compression* and the latter placement as *output compression*. In input compression, changing the volume control changes the maximum output of the hearing aid. In output controlled compression, the maximum output is not affected by the volume control setting.

All forms of compression have the goal of fitting the signal into the dynamic range of the listener, but there are different methods of reaching this goal. Compression systems may be classified as *compression limiters, slow acting volume control (AVC),* or *syllabic compressors* (Walker and Dillon 1982).

The hearing aid must have a mechanism for limiting the level of the signal that it can produce in order to maintain user comfort and safety. Very loud signals may be uncomfortable for the hearing aid user and extremely high output levels may actually cause further hearing

15

loss (Macrae 1991). Output limiting in hearing aids may be achieved by compression limiting or by peak clipping.

If a linear system is desired for all but the highest input signals, compression limiting could be implemented. Compression limiters typically have a high compression threshold (greater than 80 dB SPL), short attack and release times, and high compression ratios (greater than 5:1). Compression limiting quickly reduces the gain whenever the input level exceeds a fixed voltage (compression threshold). Dillon and Walker (1983) have recommended that output compression be used in compression limiting hearing aids. In practice, this means that in order to specify the compression threshold, the maximum power output is set below the user's loudness discomfort level. When output compression is used, setting the maximum power output automatically sets the compression threshold (compression threshold is equal to maximum output minus the gain). Compression limiting should minimize distortion in the output signal.

In contrast, in a hearing aid with peak clipping, the electrical signal is limited instantaneously at a predetermined maximum voltage, thus eliminating the peaks in the signal waveform. The maximum output level is usually set just below the listener's discomfort level. Peak clipping effectively limits the output of the hearing aid, but introduces distortion into the amplified signal. Some studies have shown decrements in speech intelligibility with peak clipping (e.g., Davis et al. 1947; Hudgins et al. 1948), whereas others have failed to show this effect (e.g., Licklider 1946). Peak clipping does affect sound quality adversely (e.g., Agnew 1988; Olsen 1991) and may actually result in a lower loudness discomfort level (Fortune and Preves 1992).

Compression may be used as an automatic volume control (AVC) to maintain a relatively constant output level, despite changes in the input level. A slow-acting compressor is used to change the gain of the amplifier as a function of long-term variations in the level of the input signal. This type of compression obviates the need of some hearing aid users to make frequent adjustments to the volume control of a linear hearing aid in order to keep the soft sounds loud enough and loud sounds tolerable. The AVC compression hearing aid automatically changes the amount of amplification applied to the signal to maintain the output of the hearing aid at the user's comfortable listening level. Slow-acting volume control compressors have a low compression threshold and longer attack and release times (release times greater than 150 msec.). The compression ratio may be high or low. Dillon and Walker (1983) recommend that input compression be used for slow acting volume control hearing aids. At present, this type of compression is rarely found in hearing aids.

Little research is available on the efficacy of slow-acting compression (AVC). Braida et al. (1979) and Dillon (1988) have indicated the potential for this form of amplification in hearing aids. King and Martin (1984) compared performance of listeners with sensorineural hearing loss with a slow-acting compression hearing aid and a linear hearing aid. Subjects preferred compression when listening to speech at normal conversational levels and higher levels. They judged the compressed signal to be quieter, more comfortable, and clearer than the uncompressed signal. Subjects also preferred compression when listening to speech in noise because the speech sounded clearer and more comfortable.

A compression hearing aid with a long release time may render inaudible low-level signals that follow an intense signal. Adaptive compression is an ingenious method of overcoming this problem. In this form of compression, the release time is dependent on the duration of the sound activating the compression circuit. For short time duration sounds, the release time is short and for long duration sounds, the release time is long (Gittles and Wilson 1987; Smriga 1987).

A different form of compression, syllabic compression, adjusts the gain of the hearing aid quickly in order to minimize variations in the level of speech within a word. Syllabic compressors have a low-compression threshold, short attack and release times, and low-compression ratios.

This type of compression is used for those hearing-impaired persons with a very narrow dynamic range. The syllabic compressor is set to fit the speech signal into the limited dynamic range of the listener by providing less amplification for the strong vowel sounds (low frequencies) and more amplification for the weaker consonant sounds (high frequencies). The purpose of using syllabic compression is to improve the intelligibility of speech, while maintaining user comfort. Syllabic compressors are used in many compression hearing aids.

A large number of studies have been done to investigate the benefit of syllabic compression in hearing aids. An extensive review is provided by Braida and his colleagues (1979). To date, research has failed to show clear-cut advantages to the use of syllabic compression systems in single-band hearing aids. Based on experiments with a two-band compression hearing aid, Moore and Glasberg (1988) have suggested that syllabic compression be used only in the high-frequency band in order to fit the signal into the limited dynamic range in that frequency region.

Recently, there has been a great deal of interest in multiband compression hearing aids. In the multiband hearing aid, the frequency range of the hearing aid is subdivided into n bands or channels (filter bands whose gain and compression characteristics may be specified according to the characteristics of the hearing aid user). Multiband compression, thus, allows different amounts of amplification and compression of the signal in different frequency regions. This is advantageous because hearing loss changes as a function of frequency as does the signal level. Theoretically, the careful selection of multiband compression characteristics will allow an almost perfect match between the dynamic range of the hearing aid user and the dynamic range of the amplified signal.

Multiband systems may be of the syllabic compression type (e.g., Villchur 1973; Barfod 1976; Abramovitz 1980; Lippman, Braida, and Durlach 1981; DeGennaro, Braida, and Durlach 1986) or the compression limiting type (e.g., Mangold and Leijon 1979; Laurence et al. 1983; Moore, Laurence, and Wright 1985; Bustamante and Braida 1987; Boothroyd et al. 1988). Slow-acting compression may also be incorporated into a multiband system (Laurence et al. 1983).

It should be noted that much of the early research on multiband compression systems was done on experimental hearing aids with many bands (up to 16). The majority of that research failed to demonstrate the superiority of multiband compression amplification over carefully chosen linear amplification systems (e.g., Abramovitz 1980; Barfod 1976; Lippman et al. 1981). It has been suggested that the failure of such multiband syllabic compression systems to improve speech intelligibility was due to the fact that independent compression in the various bands destroyed the short-term spectral cues that are important for good speech intelligibility.

Those studies showing multiband compression to be beneficial have utilized two or three bands (e.g., Villchur 1973; Laurence et al. 1983, Moore and Glasberg 1986, 1988; Moore, Glasberg, and Stone 1991; Benson, Clark, and Johnson 1992; Moore et al. 1992). Comparisons with linear hearing aids have consistently shown an advantage for the multiband systems (e.g., Moore et al. 1992). Currently there are several two- or three-band compression hearing aids available commercially. They vary in the control given the audiologist over the compression characteristics. In most of these hearing aids, the crossover frequency (frequencies) of the system can be selected by the dispenser. The compression threshold, compression ratio, and release time are other variables that may be selected (directly or indirectly) by the dispenser. A major problem in using these systems is the lack of knowledge about selection of compression parameters for hearing-impaired listeners. Some hearing aid companies have included suggested fitting procedures. None of these procedures has been experimentally validated.

Hearing aids may contain more than one type of compression. Several hearing aids utilize compression limiting on the input of the hearing aid, in addition to multiband syllabic compression. Moore and his colleagues have reported an interesting series of experiments with variations of a two-band compression system originally developed by Laurence (Laurence et al. 1983). The most recent version of the experimental hearing aid contains a dual front-end AGC system: a combination of a slow-acting compressor and a fast-acting compressor. This input compressor is used in conjunction with a two-band hearing aid with syllabic compression. Syllabic compression is used only in the high-frequency channel. This design seems promising, although it is not yet available as a commercial hearing aid.

Noise Reduction/Suppression

Many of the recent changes in hearing aid design are meant to facilitate use of the hearing aid in noisy situations. Two solutions that have been utilized in the past include the use of directional microphones and the use of high-pass filtering to reduce background noise. The directional microphone was first introduced in commercial hearing aids in 1971. The microphone is designed in a way that makes it more sensitive to sounds originating from the front of the microphone than from behind. Because the signal of interest is usually in front of the person, the directional microphone can increase the signal-to-noise ratio in many circumstances.

The amount of noise reduction achieved will depend on the amount of reverberation in the enclosure and the characteristics of the directional microphone. In an anechoic room, reduction of up to 20 dB can be measured when the signal is at 0° azimuth and the noise is at 180° azimuth for frequencies below 2000 Hz. In real rooms, Studebaker, Cox, and Formby (1980) have demonstrated that directionality decreases as the amount of reverberation increases. Nevertheless, in rooms with moderate reverberation, the directional microphone can still provide a significant improvement in signal-to-noise ratio.

Research on directional microphones has been reviewed by Mueller (1981), who concluded that listener's performance with hearing aids containing a directional microphone was superior to or equivalent to performance with an omnidirectional microphone. In a classic study, Hawkins and Yacullo (1984) evaluated the signal-to-noise ratio necessary to obtain 50% performance level on monosyllabic word materials under conditions of reverberation. Testing was done monaurally and binaurally with directional and omnidirectional microphones. The study revealed an advantage of 3 to 4 dB as the result of using a directional microphone, a 2 to 3 dB improvement as the result of binaural amplification, and an additive effect for the binaural and directional microphone advantages for the hearing-impaired listeners in environments with short and moderate reverberation times.

Despite the findings that directional microphones can be of sig-

19

nificant benefit in a variety of listening situations, directional hearing aids are used in less than 5% of hearing aid fittings (Mueller and Hawkins 1990). This is down from 20% in 1981 (Mueller 1981). Directional microphones are included in few in-the-ear model hearing aids, although it is possible to incorporate this type of microphone with beneficial results (Preves 1978).

In another method of noise suppression, a high-pass filter switch is available for use in noisy situations. When the listener is in a noisy environment, he or she can switch the filter on his or her hearing aid to one that does not amplify low-frequency energy. Because many environmental noises contain a lot of low-frequency energy, high-pass filtering can be quite effective in eliminating background noise.

A recent innovation in conventional hearing aids has been the development of hearing aids with *level dependent frequency response*. Two different approaches have been taken. Killion, Staab, and Preves (1990) have assigned the acronyms BILL (bass increases at low levels) and TILL (treble increases at low levels) to these two approaches. In the first approach, gain in the low-frequency region decreases with increases in input level. The frequency responses that would result from this type of hearing aid at low (50 dB input) and high (90 dB input) input levels appear in figure 4. This type of processing may be implemented in conventional hearing aids in several ways. Adaptive filtering may be used

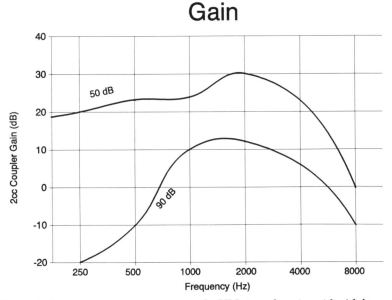

Figure 4. Frequency response curves of a BILL-type hearing aid with low- and high-input levels.

20

to suppress background noise. Either the slope of the high-pass filter can be changed according to the input level of the signal, or the cut-off frequency of the high-pass filter changes as a function of the signal level. In another method, two filters and a compression amplifier are combined in order to compress only low frequency sounds, dependent on the input level.

In the second approach, the hearing aid frequency response is a high-pass filter for low-level inputs and becomes increasingly broad-band for high levels (Killion 1990). Figure 5 illustrates the frequency responses that would result from this type of hearing aid at low (50 dB) and high (90 dB) input levels. The goal of this type of hearing aid is not noise suppression, per se, but rather the improvement of the ability to understand speech in noise.

A large number of hearing aid companies have incorporated noise suppression circuitry into their hearing aids (behind-the-ear, in-the-ear, and in-the-canal). The processing done in these new hearing aids may affect the quality of the processed signal in both positive and negative ways, just as it may improve or degrade intelligibility of the speech signal.

More sophisticated methods of noise reduction are incorporated into the digitally controlled analog and digital signal processing hearing aids. For example, the *Zeta Noise Blocker,* a hybrid integrated circuit

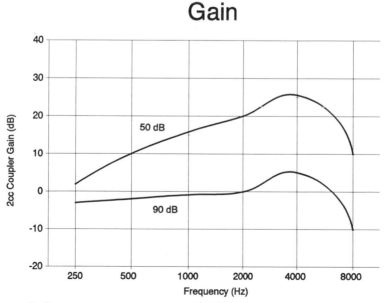

Figure 5. Frequency response curves of a TILL-type hearing aid with low- and high-input levels.

that implements a multiband adaptive filter (Graupe et al. 1986), is used in commercial hearing aids. A microprocessor is used to control a number of filters that can be adjusted and attenuated in order to suppress noise across the bandwidth of the hearing aid. The fact that processing is done across all frequencies rather than only at low frequencies differentiates the Zeta Noise Blocker from other adaptive filters used for noise suppression.

Experimental evaluations of different noise reduction hearing aids have been helpful in delineating their potential benefits. Noise reduction circuits seem to provide an improvement in speech recognition primarily when speech is presented against a background of low-frequency noise, but not when other broadband noises such as speech babble are used (e.g., Sigelman and Preves 1987; Stein and Dempesey-Hart 1984; Wolinsky 1986). This is not to say that hearing aid users do not benefit from noise reduction hearing aids. Individual differences in benefit have been found (e.g., Stach, Speerschneider, and Jerger 1987; Sigelman and Preves 1987; Dillon and Lovegrove 1993). It has been suggested that when hearing-impaired listeners do show improvements in speech recognition, release from masking and release from distortion may account for gains in speech recognition in noise (Van Tasell and Crain 1992).

Several recent studies have compared performance of listeners with several noise reduction circuits (e.g., Tyler and Kuk 1989; Schum 1990) or noise reduction approaches (Horwitz, Turner, and Fabry 1991). In general, group data have failed to reveal significant differences among noise reduction approaches in speech recognition performance. The same holds true for subjective ratings of noise-reduction hearing aids (e.g., Kuk, Tyler, and Mims 1990). However, it should be noted that in certain hearing-impaired individuals there were significant improvements (or decrements) in speech recognition as a result of different forms of processing. Subjective ratings also revealed significant preferences within individual subjects.

Bentler (1991) has obtained subjective measures of improvement on a large group of hearing aid users fit with noise reduction type hearing aids. In her study, the experimental group did not differ significantly from the control group on subjective measures. In contrast, several experimental studies have shown that listeners may prefer to listen to a signal that has been digitally processed to reduce background noise, even when improvements in speech recognition do not occur (e.g., Lim 1983; Neuman, Mills, and Schwander 1985). It has been suggested that other aspects of benefit such as fatigue, workload, and mental effort be investigated (CHABA 1989). Saunders and Levitt (1991) recently reported on the evaluation of a noise reduction technique using the measurement of reaction time in conjunction with a sentence verification task.

Digital signal processing techniques can be implemented in all-digital hearing aids. The Nicolet Phoenix hearing aid, which was available for a short period of time, incorporated a digital algorithm to achieve noise reduction and output limiting functions (Hecox and Miller 1988). The amount of noise reduction was selected individually by each subject according to his preferences. The algorithm(s) used in the digital hearing aid were proprietary and have not been revealed.

In a study utilizing the Phoenix hearing aid (Roeser and Taylor 1988), performance with the digital hearing aid using frequency shaping alone was compared with performance using frequency shaping plus the digital noise reduction algorithm. Addition of the noise reduction algorithm was reported to yield significant increases in speech recognition scores (Northwestern University Auditory Test No. 6) for speech presented in speech spectrum shaped noise (12 dB S/N).

Methods of Reducing Acoustic Feedback. Acoustic feedback is a special problem in hearing aids that contain a substantial amount of gain, hearing aids that are used in conjunction with vented or open molds, and in-the-ear hearing aids. The simplest solutions to the feedback problem have involved separation of the microphone and receiver in order to minimize the pickup of leaked sound (e.g., utilization of an ear level receiver in conjunction with a bodyworn microphone, or placement of the microphone on one ear and the receiver on the opposite ear in a CROS fitting). Earmold modifications are often used to minimize feedback. Placement of damping materials in the tubing and modifications to the earmold bore are two ways of suppressing feedback. Use of soft earmold materials and deep insertion of the earmold are other techniques. Reduction of the gain in the hearing aid and modification of the high-frequency response are commonly used methods that are successful in reducing feedback, but may limit the benefit of the hearing aid. Electronic methods such as use of negative feedback in the amplifier (Preves, Sigelman, and LeMay 1986) and phase compensation in the amplifier (Egolf 1982) have been suggested as methods to suppress feedback.

The newest method to be implemented in a digital hearing aid is adaptive feedback cancellation (Bisgaard and Dyrlund 1991). Feedback cancellation in this hearing aid is implemented by injecting a low-level noise signal into the acoustic signal path. The characteristics of the feedback path are determined using a correlation technique. The feedback path is then simulated within the hearing aid using an adaptive filter. The acoustic signal is filtered through this simulated feedback

23

path and subtracted from the input to the hearing aid to cancel the actual feedback. This process may allow up to 10 dB of additional gain in the hearing aid.

INTERFACING THE HEARING AID AND ASSISTIVE DEVICES

Although noise reduction circuitry in wearable hearing aids has failed to yield substantial improvements in speech recognition, assistive listening devices (e.g., frequency modulation and infrared listening systems, as well as induction loops) are very effective in improving the signal-to-noise ratio. In these systems, the microphone of the hearing aid is placed directly in front of the signal of interest to the listener, thus, the signal-to-noise ratio is optimized and the degradation of reverberation is avoided. Coupling of the personal hearing aid to these assistive devices is accomplished by use of inductive coupling (neckloop or silhouette inductor) or by direct audio input (see Compton 1989, for a comprehensive treatment of assistive listening devices).

Inductive coupling can be used when the hearing aid user has a telecoil in his personal hearing aid. Originally, the telecoil was included in the hearing aid in order to facilitate use by the hearing aid user of the telephone. But the telecoil also allows access to assistive listening devices. With the passage of the Americans with Disabilities Act (ADA), more and more public facilities are providing assistive listening systems (large area listening systems). But only 10 to 30 percent of hearing aids include a telecoil (Cranmer-Briskey 1992b). In part, this may be due to the prevalence of in-the-ear hearing aids. The limited space available in in-the-ear aids may require that the telecoil be small. Because the telecoil is magnetic wire with a large number of turns, the strength of the telecoil is related to its size. The development of amplified telecoils makes it possible to include a more powerful telecoil in in-the-ear aids (Cranmer-Briskey 1992b). The recommendation of a telecoil in the hearing aid and education of hearing aid users in its use can result in substantial improvements in hearing aid use in many difficult listening situations.

When hearing aids are coupled to assistive listening systems inductively, the frequency response of the hearing aid may change (e.g., Hawkins and Schum 1985; Thibodeau, McCaffrey, and Abrahamson 1988). Measurement protocols have been developed to ascertain the effects of such coupling (Hawkins 1987a,b; Lewis, Feigin, and Stelmachowicz 1991). Measures of listener performance with the inductive coupling should also be ascertained.

Direct electrical input of the signal to the hearing aid is an alternative method of improving signal-to-noise ratio. Direct audio input

(DAI) is accomplished through an attachment to the hearing aid (the audio shoe). This option is most commonly available in behind-the-ear aids, but can also be implemented in some in-the-ear and body aids. When using direct audio input, the electroacoustic characteristics of the hearing aid may be different than when the DAI is in use. Measurements of performance of the hearing aid in the DAI mode should be made (e.g., Hawkins 1987a).

RECENT DEVELOPMENTS IN
MEASUREMENTS OF HEARING AID PERFORMANCE

Many of the newer hearing aids contain some form of nonlinear processing (e.g., adaptive frequency response, full-range compression, multiband compression, noise suppression). The frequency response of these hearing aids changes as a function of input level. In fact, even linear hearing aids become nonlinear at high-input levels. The importance of determining the effect of the hearing aid at multiple input levels has, thus, been emphasized with regard to both subjective and objective measures. Villchur (1982) has emphasized the need to use speech materials that vary in level when evaluating performance with a compression hearing aid. This may be accomplished by testing at multiple input levels or by using speech materials that include normal variations in level.

An evaluation of the electroacoustic characteristics of nonlinear hearing aids also requires the use of multiple input levels. In addition, a different type of test signal is necessary. An adequate representation of the frequency response and maximum output of a linear hearing aid can be obtained using swept pure-tones. In a nonlinear hearing aid, however, use of a swept pure-tone signal results in an inflated measure of the gain in the low frequencies, a measurement artifact called *blooming*. This problem in the measurement of compression systems has been known for some time. However, the ANSI recommended procedure (ANSI Standard S3.22-1987) for measuring the frequency response of hearing aids is primarily concerned with measuring the frequency response for aids in linear operation (whether the hearing aid be of the linear or compression type). In order to characterize the performance of a nonlinear hearing aid used in the nonlinear mode accurately, however, alternate measurement procedures are necessary. It is for this reason that a new ANSI standard has been developed and adopted (ANSI S34.2-1992) that specifies use of a broad-band noise signal to measure the input-output function of hearing aids. Use of a complex signal gives a more accurate representation of the frequency response of the system for complex signals like speech. The measures are made at several input levels in order to ascertain the input-output characteristics of the hearing aid system. The new standard specifies the characteristics of the noise to be used as the test signal, the long-term spectrum of the noise, the method of analysis to be used, and the multiple input levels to be used for specifying the input-output characteristics of the hearing aid.

Recently, probe-microphone real-ear measurements have become an important adjunct to the fitting of hearing aids. In many cases, the real-ear measurement system is used to check that the hearing aid is achieving the goals of a particular prescriptive hearing aid procedure (i.e., real ear insertion gain). The probe microphone can also be used to measure output levels in the ear (i.e., real ear saturation response), to determine the output level as a function of frequency with a given input and volume control setting (i.e., real ear aided response), to ascertain distortion in the hearing aid, and to facilitate the adjustment of programmable hearing aids. It can also be used to assess performance of telecoils with a signal from the telephone, directional microphone, assistive listening devices, and the occlusion effect caused by the hearing aid or earmold. An extensive discussion of probe microphone measurement procedures and applications is provided by Mueller, Hawkins, and Northern (1992).

TECHNOLOGY AND IMPLEMENTATION
OF FITTING PROCEDURES

One of the variables that should be included in the calculation of target coupler (full-on) gain values is the amount of reserve gain needed and the correction for differences between real ear and coupler measures (CORFIG, e.g., Killion and Monser 1980). Various prescriptive procedures will differ with regard to reserve gain. This information is readily available. Average coupler-to-real-ear correction values will differ depending on the hearing aid style and microphone location. Tables of CORFIG values are available (e.g., Skinner 1988; Bentler and Pavlovic 1989; Hawkins 1992). Computer-based hearing aid fitting systems simplify the calculation of 2cc full-on gain and SSPL90 values by incorporating these corrections into the software (e.g., Revit 1990; Valente, Valente, and Vass 1991; Dillon, Byrne, and Battaglia 1992).

CORFIG values are corrections for the average ear. However, it is preferable to individualize the real-ear correction. This may be particularly crucial in the case of young children with very small ear canal volumes. Procedures for individualizing the CORFIG using probe microphone measurements have been proposed (e.g., Punch, Chi, and Patterson 1990). An extensive discussion of this issue is provided by Mueller (1992).

26

CONCLUSIONS

The major changes in hearing aids over the past ten years have been the increased miniaturization of hearing aids and the introduction of digitally controlled analog and digital signal-processing hearing aids. Many of the new hearing aids include alternatives to linear amplification; e.g., automatic signal processing, level-dependent frequency response, and multiband compression. The major changes in hearing aid measurement are the development of real ear measurement systems and the specification of a new method for measuring the electroacoustic characteristics of hearing aids.

Miniaturization has resulted in the widespread use of in-the-ear hearing aids for all but those with profound hearing loss. Many of the limitations of older generation in-the-ear hearing aids have been overcome. Virtually anything that can be done in a behind-the-ear aid is now possible in an in-the-ear aid (with the exception of digital signal-processing technology). For example, flexibility in shaping the frequency response is available in programmable hearing aids. Amplification options such as multiple frequency responses and multiband compression amplification are now also available. The development of preamplifiers for induction circuits and the increased availability of assistive listening devices in public places will, we hope, result in increased availability of the induction coil in in-the-ear aids.

The application of digital technology to hearing aids has resulted in extremely versatile instruments. The dispenser has more control over electroacoustic characteristics of the hearing aid than was ever possible before. With progammable hearing aids a dispenser can often obtain a better match to the desired frequency response than with standard circuitry. Both the frequency response and output levels of programmable hearing aids may be adjusted to compensate for changes in hearing or to maximize the quality and comfort of the hearing aid user. This makes the hearing aid fitting an ongoing process and can result in greater user satisfaction. Multiband systems may be particularly helpful in the adjustment of maximum output for those hearing aid users whose loudness discomfort levels differ as a function of frequency.

There are also more choices to make about the type of amplification to be used. In the past, the majority of hearing aids were linear amplifiers. Output limiting was achieved with peak clipping. This meant the specification of only two parameters: the frequency-gain response and the maximum output level. Advances in prescriptive fitting procedures made hearing aid selection relatively easy for many clinicians. However, now a dispenser has to decide among linear hearing aids with a single setting, single-channel compression hearing aids, multiband compression hearing aids, hearing aids with multiple frequency responses, or hearing aids with level-dependent frequency responses.

User-related criteria for deciding when to use a particular type of hearing aid have not yet been developed. Technological changes in hearing aids have resulted in many ways to fit the signal into the listener's dynamic range. This may be achieved by using compression limiting, wide dynamic range compression, or other forms of level-dependent frequency response. It has been recommended that compression be used when the dynamic range is less than 40 dB (e.g., Skinner 1988). At present, however, compression limiting is probably the only form of compression for which there is agreement on how to set the compression parameters. Prescriptive procedures for wide dynamic range systems are still being developed (e.g., Moore 1987).

With regard to the choice of multimemory versus level- dependent frequency response hearing aids, the choice is unclear. Both types of hearing aids may be used to provide different frequency responses with change in input level. Which type is more beneficial? In the first type, the user determines when a change in frequency response is necessary. The change is accomplished with either a remote control or a control on the hearing aid case. Changes occur automatically in the hearing aid with level-dependent frequency response. It is possible that there are user-related characteristics that would make one approach superior to the other. But, because these hearing aids are relatively new, studies comparing the two approaches are unavailable.

Research with experimental hearing aids has consistently shown benefit for some listeners, but not for others. In the past, the hearing aid circuits available were those that could be expected to show benefit for large groups of hearing aid users. With the increased capability to customize hearing aids with programmable linear and compression hearing aids, there is a need to develop diagnostic tests to identify the underlying characteristics of hearing loss that would predict benefit from a particular combination of processing schemes. Prescriptive fitting procedures have provided a theoretical framework for the choice of linear amplification. It is hoped that the proliferation of nonlinear amplification systems will provide the impetus for the development of prescriptive procedures for these systems.

Real-ear measurement systems have become an important tool in the fitting of linear hearing aids and should be equally helpful in setting the parameters of nonlinear amplification. Real-ear measurements are most often used to verify that the objectives of a prescriptive fitting procedure (frequency-gain response and maximum output level) have been met. Alternative measures made with various input levels can give information about the placement of the amplified speech spectrum in relation to threshold and loudness discomfort (real ear aided response). This type of measure would be particularly useful in understanding what a nonlinear hearing aid will do to a speech signal for a particular hearing aid user. When measuring nonlinear amplification systems a broadband signal should be used. The broadband stimulus specified in the ANSI Standard (S34.2-1992) would be equally applicable to measurement with real-ear measurement systems.

REFERENCES

Abramovitz, R. 1980. Frequency shaping and multiband compression in hearing aids. *Journal of Communication Disorders* 13:483–88.

Agnew, G. 1988. Hearing instrument distortion: What does it mean for the listener? *Hearing Instruments* 39(10):10–20.

American National Standards Institute. 1987. *Specification of Hearing Aid Characteristics.* ANSI S3.22–1987. New York: American National Standards Institute, Inc.

American National Standards Institute. 1992. *Testing Hearing Aids with a Broad Band Noise Signal.* ANSI S3.42–1992. New York: American National Standards Institute, Inc.

Amerine, K. L. 1992. Software leads the way for programmable compatibility. *Hearing Instruments* 13(10):20 23.

Barfod, J. 1976. *Multichannel Compression Hearing Aids: Effects of Recruitment on Speech Intelligibility.* The Acoustics Laboratory, Technical Univ. of Denmark, Report No. 11.

Benson, D., Clark, T. M., and Johnson, J. S. 1992. Patient experiences with multiband full dynamic range compression. *Ear and Hearing* 13.320–30.

Bentler, R. A. 1991. Clinical implications and limitations of current noise reduction circuitry. In *The Vanderbilt Hearing Aid Report II,* eds. G. A. Studebaker, F. H. Bess, and L. B. Beck. Parkton, MD: York Press, Inc.

Bentler, R. A., and Pavlovic, C. V. 1989. Transfer functions and correction factors used in hearing aid evaluation and research. *Ear and Hearing* 10:58–63.

Berger, K. W., Abel, D. B., Hagberg, E. N., Puzz, L. A., Varavvas, D. M., and Weldele, F. J. 1982. Successes and problems of hearing aid users. *Hearing Aid Journal* 35 (11):26–30.

Bergman, M. 1971. Hearing and aging: Implications of recent research findings. *Audiology* 10:164–71.

Bergman, M., Blumenfeld, V., Cascardo, D., Dash, B., Levitt, H., and Margulies, M. 1976. Age-related decrement in hearing for speech: Sampling and longitudinal studies. *Journal of Gerontology* 31:533–38.

Bisgaard, N., and Dyrlund 1991. Acoustic feedback Part 2: A digital system for suppression of feedback. *Hearing Instruments* 42(10):44–46.

Bisgaard, N., Christiansen, C., and Morrison, P. 1993. A universal interface for programmable hearing instruments. *Hearing Instruments* 44(1):14–17.

Boothroyd, A., Springer, N., Smith, L., and Schulman, J. 1988. Amplitude compression and profound hearing loss. *Journal of Speech and Hearing Research* 31: 362–76.

Braida, L. D., Durlach, N. I., Lippmann, R. P., Hicks, B. L., Rabinowitz, W. M., and Reed, C. M. 1979. *Hearing Aids—A Review of Past Research of Linear Amplification, Amplitude Compression and Frequency Lowering.* ASHA

Monograph #19. Rockville, MD: American Speech-Language-Hearing Association.

Branderbit, P. L. 1991. A standardized programming system and three-channel compression hearing instrument technology. *Hearing Instruments* 42(1):24–30.

Bustamante, D. K. and Braida, L. D. 1987. Multiband compression limiting for hearing-impaired listeners. *Journal of Rehabilitation Research and Development* 24(4):149–60.

Carhart, R., and Tillman, T. W. 1970. Interaction of competing speech signals with hearing loss. *Archives of Otolaryngology* 91:273–79.

CHABA 1989. *Removal of Noise from Noise-degraded Speech Signals.* (Report of the) Committee on Hearing, Bioacoustics and Biomechanics, Commission on Behavioral and Social Sciences and Education, National Research Council. Washington, DC: National Academy Press.

Compton, C. L. 1989. Assistive devices. *Seminars in Hearing* 10(1).

Cranmer-Briskey, K. 1992a. 1992 *Hearing Instruments* Dispenser Survey results. *Hearing Instruments* 43:8–15.

Cranmer-Briskey, K. 1992b. The ADA spells urgency for telecoil use. *Hearing Instruments* 43(8):8–12.

Cummins, K. L., and Hecox, K. E. 1987. Ambulatory testing of digital hearing aid algorithms. In *Proceedings of the 10th Annual Conference on Rehabilitation Technology,* eds. R. D. Steele and W. Gerrety. Washington, D.C.: RESNA-Association for the Advancement of Rehabilitation Technology.

Davis, H., Stevens, S. S., Nichols, Jr., R. H., Hudgins, C. V., Marquis, R. J., Peterson, G. E., and Ross, D. A. 1947. *Hearing Aids: An Experimental Study of Design Objectives.* Cambridge, MA: Harvard University Press.

DeGennaro S. V., Braida, L. D., and Durlach, N. I. 1986. Multichannel syllabic compression for severely impaired listeners. *Journal of Rehabilitation Research and Development* 23:17–24.

Dillon, H. 1988. Compression in Hearing Aids. In *Handbook of Hearing Aid Amplification,* Volume I, ed. R. E. Sandlin. Boston, MA: College-Hill Press.

Dillon, H., Byrne, D., and Battaglia, J. 1992. Hearing instrument selection: By dispenser or by computer. *Hearing Instruments* 43(8):18–21.

Dillon, H., and Lovegrove, R. 1993. Single-microphone noise reduction systems for hearing aids: A review and an evaluation. In *Acoustical Factors Affecting Hearing Aid Performance,* eds. G. A. Studebaker and I. Hochberg. Needham Heights, MA: Allyn and Bacon.

Dillon, H., and Walker, G. 1983. Compression—input or output control? *Hearing Instruments* 34(9):20–22, 42.

Dirks, D., Morgan, D. E., and Dubno, J. R. 1982. A procedure for quantifying the effects of noise on speech recognition. *Journal of Speech and Hearing Disorders* 47:114–23.

Dubno, J. R., Dirks, D. D., and Morgan, D. E. 1984. Effects of age and mild hearing loss on speech recognition in noise. *Journal of the Acoustical Society of America* 76:87–96.

Egolf, D. P. 1982. Review of the acoustic feedback literature from a control systems point of view. In *The Vanderbilt Hearing Aid Report,* eds. G. A. Studebaker and F. H. Bess. Upper Darby, Pa.: Monographs in Contemporary Audiology.

Engebretsen, A. M., Morley, R. E., and O'Connell, M. P. 1986. A wearable, pocket-sized processor for digital hearing aid and other hearing prosthesis applications. *Proceedings of the International Conference on Acoustics, Speech and*

Signal Processing. (ICASSP-1986), Institute of Electrical and Electronic Engineering.

Engebretsen, A. M., Morley, R. E., and Popelka, G. R. 1987. Development of an ear-level digital hearing aid and computer-assisted fitting procedure. *Journal of Rehabilitation Research and Development* 24(4):55–64.

Finitzo-Hieber, T., and Tillman, T. W. 1978. Room acoustics effects on monosyllabic word discrimination ability for normal and hearing-impaired children. *Journal of Speech and Hearing Research* 21:440–58.

Florentine, M., Buus, S., Scharf, B., and Zwicker, E. 1980. Frequency selectivity in normally-hearing and hearing-impaired observers. *Journal of Speech and Hearing Research* 23:646–69.

Fortune, T., and Preves, D. A. 1992. Hearing aid saturation and aided loudness discomfort. *Journal of Speech and Hearing Research* 35:175–85.

Gengel, R. W. 1971. Acceptable speech-to-noise ratios for aided speech discrimination by the hearing-impaired. *Journal of Auditory Research* 11:219–22.

Gittles, T. and Wilson, F. A. 1987. Compression amplification with environment controlled release time. *Hearing Instruments* 38:39–41.

Graupe, D., and Causey, D. 1975. Development of a hearing aid system with independently adjustable subranges of its spectrum using microprocessor hardware. *Bulletin of Prosthetic Research* 12:241–42.

Graupe, D., Grosspietsch, J. K., and Basseas, S. P. 1987. A single-microphone based self-adaptive filter of noise from speech and its performance evaluation. *Journal of Rehabilitation Research and Development* 24(4):119–26.

Graupe, D., Grosspietsch, J. K., and Taylor R. 1986. A self adaptive noise filtering system. Part 1: Overview and description. *Hearing Instruments* 37:29–34.

Hawkins, D. B. 1987a. Assessment of FM systems with an ear canal probe tube microphone system. *Ear and Hearing* 8:301–3.

Hawkins, D. B. 1987a. Clinical ear canal probe tube measurements. *Ear and Hearing* 8 (5S), 74S 81S.

Hawkins, D. B. 1992. Corrections and transformations relevant to hearing aid selection. In *Probe Microphone Measurement Hearing Aid Selection and Assessment*, eds. H. G. Mueller, D. B. Hawkins and J. L. Northern. San Diego, CA: Singular Publishing Group, Inc.

Hawkins, D. B., and Schum, D. J. 1985. Some effects of FM coupling on hearing aid characteristics. *Journal of Speech and Hearing Disorders* 50:132 41.

Hawkins, D. B., and Yacullo, W. S. 1984. Signal-to-noise ratio advantage of binaural hearing aids and directional microphones under different levels of reverberation. *Journal of Speech and Hearing Disorders* 49:278–86.

Hearing Instruments 1992. Dispenser programmable hearing instruments update. *Hearing Instruments* 43(9):6–26.

Hecox, K. E. 1988. Evaluation of hearing aid performance. *Seminars in Hearing* 9(3):239–51.

Hecox, K. E., and Miller, E. 1988. New hearing instrument technologies. *Hearing Instruments* 39(3):38–40.

Hecox, K. E., and Punch, J. L. 1988. The impact of digital technology on the selection and fitting of hearing aids. *The American Journal of Otology* 9(Suppl.): 77–85.

Horwitz, A. R., Turner, C. W., and Fabry, D. A. 1991. Effects of different frequency response strategies upon recognition and preference for audible speech stimuli. *Journal of Speech and Hearing Research* 34:1185–96.

Hudgins, C., Marquis, R., Nichols, R., Peterson, G., and Ross, D. 1948. The comparative performance of an experimental hearing aid and two commercial instruments. *Journal of the Acoustical Society of America* 20:241–58.

Keith, R. W., and Talis, H. P. 1972. The effects of white noise on PB scores of normal-hearing and hearing-impaired listeners. *Audiology* 11:177–86.

Killion, M. C. 1990. A high fidelity hearing aid. *Hearing Instruments* 41(8): 38–39.

Killion, M. C. 1981. Earmold options for wideband hearing aids. *Journal of Speech and Hearing Research* 46:10–20.

Killion, M. C. 1982. Transducers, earmolds and sound quality considerations. In *The Vanderbilt Hearing Aid Report*, eds. G. A. Studebaker and F. H. Bess. Upper Darby, PA: Monographs in Contemporary Audiology.

Killion, M. C. 1993. Transducers and acoustic couplings: The hearing aid problem that is (mostly) solved. In *Acoustical Factors Affecting Hearing Aid Performance* (second edition), eds. G. A. Studebaker and I. Hochberg. Needham Heights, MA: Allyn and Bacon.

Killion, M. C., Berlin, C., and Hood, L. 1984. A low frequency emphasis open canal hearing aid. *Hearing Instruments* 35(8):30–34.

Killion, M. C., and Monser, E. 1980. CORFIG: Coupler responses for flat insertion gain. In *Acoustical Factors Affecting Hearing Aid Performance*, eds. G. A. Studebaker and I. Hochberg. Baltimore, MD: University Park Press.

Killion, M. C., Staab, W. J., and Preves, D. A. 1990. Classifying automatic signal processors. *Hearing Instruments* 41(8):24, 26.

King, A. B., and Martin, M. C. 1984. Is AGC beneficial in hearing aids. *British Journal of Audiology* 18:31–38.

Kuk, F. K., Tyler, R. S., and Mims, L. 1990. Subjective ratings of noise-reduction hearing aids. *Scandinavian Audiology* 19:237–44.

Laurence, R., Moore, B., and Glasberg, B. 1983. A comparison of behind-the-ear high-fidelity linear hearing aids and two-channel compression aids in the laboratory and in everyday life. *British Journal of Audiology* 17:31–48.

Leshowitz, B. 1977. Speech intelligibility in noise for listeners with sensorineural hearing damage. Final Papers Report of the Institute for Perception Research. Eindhoven, The Netherlands.

Leshowitz, B., and Lindstrom, R. 1977. Measurement of nonlinearities in listeners with sensorineural hearing loss. In *Psychophysics and Physiology in Hearing*, eds. E. F. Evans and J. P. Wilson. London: Academic Press.

Levitt, H. 1982. An array-processor, computer hearing aid. Presented at the Annual convention of the American Speech-Language-Hearing Association, Toronto.

Levitt, H., Neuman, A., Mills, R., and Schwander, T. 1986. A digital master hearing aid. *Journal of Rehabilitation Research and Development* 23(1):79–87.

Lewis, D., Feigin, J., and Stelmachowicz, P. 1991. Evaluation and assessment of FM systems. *Ear and Hearing* 12:268–80.

Licklider, J. 1946 Effects of amplitude distortion upon the intelligibility of speech. *Journal of the Acoustical Society of America* 18:429–34.

Lim, J.S. 1983. *Speech Enhancement*. Englewood Cliffs, NJ: Prentice Hall.

Lippman, R., Braida, L., and Durlach, N.I. 1981. Study of multichannel amplitude compression and linear amplification for persons with sensorineural hearing loss. *Journal of the Acoustical Society of America* 69:524–34.

Macrae, J. 1991. Permanent threshold shift associated with overamplification by hearing aids. *Journal of Speech and Hearing Research* 34:403–14.

Mangold, S., and Leijon, A. 1979. A programmable hearing aid with multi-channel compression. *Scandinavian Audiology* 8:121–26.

Moore, B. C. 1987. Design and evaluation of a two-channel compression hearing aid. *Journal of Rehabilitation Research and Development* 24(4):181–92.

Moore, B. C., and Glasberg, B. R. 1988. A comparison of four methods of implementing automatic gain control (AGC) in hearing aids. *British Journal of Audiology* 22:93–104.

Moore, B. C., and Glasberg, B. R. 1986. A comparison of two-channel and single-channel compression hearing aids. *Audiology* 25:210–26.

Moore, B. C., Glasberg, B. R., and Stone, M. A. 1991. Optimization of a slow-acting automatic gain control system for use in hearing aids. *British Journal of Audiology* 25:171–82.

Moore, B. C., Johnson, J. S., Clark, T. M., and Pluvinage, V. 1992. Evaluation of a dual-channel full dynamic range compression system for people with sensorineural hearing loss. *Ear and Hearing* 13:349–70.

Moore, B. C., Laurence, R. F., and Wright, D. 1985. Improvements in speech intelligibility in quiet and in noise produced by two-channel compression hearing aids. *British Journal of Audiology* 19:175–87.

Mueller, H. G. 1981. Directional microphone hearing aids: A 10 year report. *Hearing Instruments* 32(11):18–20, 66.

Mueller, H. G. 1992. Individualizing the ordering of custom hearing aids. In *Probe Microphone Measurements Hearing Aid Selection and Assessment*, eds. H. G. Mueller, D. B. Hawkins, and J. L. Northern. San Diego, CA: Singular Publishing Group, Inc.

Mueller, H. G., and Hawkins, D. B. 1990. Three important considerations in hearing aid selection. In *Handbook of Hearing Aid Amplification*, Volume II, ed. R. E. Sandlin. Boston, MA: College-Hill Press.

Mueller, H. G., Hawkins, D. B., and Northern, J. L. 1992. *Probe Microphone Measurements Hearing Aid Selection and Assessment*. San Diego, CA: Singular Publishing Group, Inc.

Nabelek, A. K., and Mason, D. 1981. Effect of noise and reverberation on binaural and monaural word identification by subjects with various audiograms. *Journal of Speech and Hearing Research* 24:375–83.

Nabelek, A. K., and Pickett, J. M. 1974a. Monaural and binaural speech perception through hearing aids under noise and reverberation with normal and hearing-impaired listeners. *Journal of Speech and Hearing Research* 17:724–39.

Nabelek, A. K., and Pickett, J. M. 1974b. Reception of consonants in a classroom as affected by monaural and binaural listening, noise, reverberation, and hearing aids. *Journal of the Acoustical Society of America* 56:628–39.

Nabelek, I. V., Koike, K. J. M., and Wood, W. S. 1981. Intelligibility of speech with reverberation and amplitude compression. *Journal of the Acoustical Society of America* 69:S97.

Neuman, A. C., Mills, R., and Schwander, T. 1985. Noise reduction: Effects on consonant perception by normal hearing listeners. Paper presented at the Annual Convention of the American Speech-Language-Hearing Association, Washington, D.C.

Nunley, J., Staab, W., Steadman, J., Wechsler, P., and Spencer, B. 1983. A wearable digital hearing aid. *The Hearing Journal* 10:29–31, 34–35.

Olsen, W. O. 1991. Clinical assessment of output limiting and speech enhancement techniques. In *The Vanderbilt Hearing Aid Report II*, eds. G. A. Studebaker, F. H. Bess, and L. B. Beck. Parkton, MD: York Press.

Pearsons, K. S., Bennett, R. L., and Fidell, S. 1976. Speech levels in various environments. *Report No. 3281*. Cambridge, MA: Bolt Beranek and Newman, Inc.

Pick, G. F., Evans, E. F., and Wilson, J. P. 1977. Frequency resolution in patients with hearing loss of cochlear origin. In *Psychophysics and Physiology of Hearing*, eds. E. F. Evans and J. P. Wilson. London: Academic Press.

Plomp, R. 1978. Auditory handicap of hearing impairment and the limited benefit of hearing aids. *Journal of the Acoustical Society of America* 63:533–49.

Plomp, R. 1988. The negative effect of amplitude compression in multichannel hearing aids in the light of the modulation-transfer function. *Journal of the Acoustical Society of America* 83:2322–27.

Preves, D. A. 1978. Directivity of in-the-ear aids with nondirectional and directional microphones. *Hearing Aid Journal* 29:6.

Preves, D. A. 1988. Principles of signal processing. In *Handbook of Hearing Aid Amplification*, Volume 1, ed. R. E. Sandlin. Boston: College-Hill Press.

Preves, D. A., Sigelman, J. A., and LeMay, P. R. 1986. A feedback stabilizing circuit for hearing aids. *Hearing Instruments* 37(4):34–40,51.

Punch, J. L., and Beck, E. L. 1980. Low frequency response of hearing aids and judgments of aided speech quality. *Journal of Speech and Hearing Disorders* 45:325–35.

Punch, J. L., and Beck, L. B. 1986. Relative effects of low-frequency amplification on syllable recognition and speech quality. *Ear and Hearing* 7:57–62.

Punch, J., Chi, C., and Patterson, J. 1990. A recommended protocol for prescriptive use of target gain rules. *Hearing Instruments* 41(4):12–19.

Revit, L. 1990. A software program for calculating 2cc full on gain and SSPL90 targets. *Hearing Instruments* 41(4): 34–35.

Roeser, R. J., and Taylor, K. 1988. Audiometric and field testing with a digital hearing instrument. *Hearing Instruments* 39(4):14–22.

Saunders, G. H., and Levitt, H. 1991. An automated true-false reaction-time test for evaluating noise-reduction systems. Paper presented at the convention of the American Speech-Language-Hearing Association Convention, Atlanta.

Schum, D.J. 1990. Noise reduction strategies for elderly, hearing-impaired listeners. *Journal of American Academy of Audiology* 1:31–36.

Schwartz, D. M., Surr, R. K., Montgomery, A. A., Prosek, R. A., and Walden, B. E. 1979. Performance of high frequency impaired listeners with conventional and extended high frequency amplification. *Audiology* 18: 157–74.

Sigelman, J., and Preves, D. A. 1987. Field trials of a new adaptive signal processor hearing aid circuit. *The Hearing Journal* 40(4):24–29.

Skafte, M.D. 1988. Hearing health care market in the 1980's. Hearing instrument market—1988. *Hearing Instruments* 39(5):4–12.

Skinner, M. W. 1980. Speech intelligibility in noise-induced hearing loss: Effects of high frequency amplification. *Journal of the Acoustical Society of America* 67:306–17.

Skinner, M. W. 1988. *Hearing Aid Evaluation*. Englewood Cliffs, NJ: Prentice Hall.

Skinner, M. W., and Miller, J. 1983. Amplification bandwidth and intelligibility of speech in quiet and noise for listeners with sensorineural hearing loss. *Audiology* 22:253–79.

Skinner, M. W., Karstaedt, M. M., and Miller, J. D. 1982. Amplification bandwidth and speech intelligibility for two listeners with sensorineural hearing loss. *Audiology* 21:251–68.

Smriga, D. J. 1987. Improving speech perception in noise: the frequency domain and the intensity domain. *Hearing Instruments* 38:18–21.

Stach, B. A., Speerschneider, J. M., and Jerger, J.,F. 1987. Evaluating the efficacy of automatic signal processing hearing aids. *The Hearing Journal* 40(3):15–19.

Stein, L., and Dempesey-Hart, D. 1984. Listener-assessed intelligibility of a hearing aid self-adaptive noise filter. *Ear and Hearing* 5:199–204.

Studebaker, G. A., Cox, R. M., and Formby, C. 1980. The effect of environment on the directional performance of head-worn hearing aids. In *Acoustical Factors Affecting Hearing Aid Performance*, eds. G. A. Studebaker and I. Hochberg. Baltimore: University Park Press.

Sullivan, J. A., Allsman, C. S., Nielsen, L. B., and Mobley, J. P. 1992. Amplification for listeners with steeply sloping, high-frequency hearing loss. *Ear and Hearing* 13:35–45.

Tecca, J., and Goldstein, D. 1984. Effect of low frequency hearing aid response on four measures of speech perception. *Ear and Hearing* 5:22–29.

Thibodeau, L., McCaffrey, H., and Abrahamson, J. 1988. Effects of coupling hearing aids to FM systems via neckloops. *Journal of the Academy of Rehabilitation Audiology* 21:49–56.

Tillman, T. W., Carhart, R., and Olsen, W. O. 1970. Hearing aid efficiency in a competing speech situation. *Journal of Speech and Hearing Research* 13:789–811.

Tyler, R. S., and Kuk, F. K. 1989. The effects of "noise suppression" hearing aids on consonant recognition in speech-babble and low-frequency noise. *Ear and Hearing* 10:243–49.

Tyler, R. S., and Summerfield, A. Q. 1980. Psychoacoustical and phoentic measures of temporal processing in normal and hearing-impaired listeners. In *Psychophysical, Physiological, and Behavioral Studies of Hearing*, eds. G. Van den Brink and F. A. Bilsen. Delft, The Netherlands: Delft University Press.

Tyler, R. S., Fernandes, M., and Wood, E. J. 1980. Masking, temporal integration and speech intelligibility in individuals with noise-induced hearing loss. In *Disorders of Auditory Function*. Volume III, eds. I. G. Taylor and A. Markides. London: Academic Press.

United States Bureau of the Census 1990. *Census of Population. General Population Characteristics.* Washington, DC: U.S. Government Printing Office.

Valente, M., Valente, M., and Vass, W. 1990. Selecting and appropriate matrix for ITE/ITC hearing instruments. *Hearing Instruments* 41(4):20–24.

Van Tassell, D. J., and Crain, T. R. 1992. Noise reduction hearing aids: Release from masking and release from distortion. *Ear and Hearing* 13:114–21.

Villchur, E. 1973. Signal processing to improve speech intelligibility in perceptive deafness. *Journal of the Acoustical Society of America* 53:1646–57.

Villchur, E. 1982. The evaluation of amplitude-compression processing for hearing aids. In *The Vanderbilt Hearing Aid Report*, eds. G. A. Studebaker and F. H. Bess. Upper Darby, PA: Monographs in Contemporary Audiology.

Waldhauer, F., and Villchur, E. 1988 Full dynamic range multiband compression in a hearing aid. *Hearing Journal* 41(9):29–32.

Walker, G., and Dillon, H. 1982. *Compression in Hearing Aids: An Analysis, a Review, and Some Recommendations* (Report No. 90). Sydney, Australia: National Acoustics Laboratories.

Widin, G. P., and Mangold, S. 1988. Fitting a programmable hearing instrument. *Hearing Instruments* 39(6):38–41,54.

Williamson, M. J., and Punch, J. L. 1990. Speech enhancement in digital hearing aids. *Seminars in Hearing* 11(1):68–78.

Wolinsky, S. 1986. Clinical assessment of a self-adaptive noise filtering system. *The Hearing Journal* 39:29–32.

INDEX

37

Direct audio input (DAI), 24
Direct electrical input of signal to hearing aid, 24–25
Directional hearing aids and microphones, 19–20
Distortion, 2, 3; at high frequencies, 13
Dynamic range: reduced, 2; signal to fit listener's, 28

Earmold: feedback control and, 23; sound leakage from, 3
Electret microphone, 13
Eyeglass hearing aid, 11

Feedback. *See* Acoustic feedback
Filter configuration, obtaining optimal, 13
Filtering, 12–19; adaptive, 20–21; digital logic to change type of, 9; high-pass, 19, 20
Fitting procedures, 26
Frequency, differential amplification as a function of, 12
Frequency modulation systems, 24
Frequency response hearing aid, multimemory vs. level-dependent, 28
Frequency responses: ANSI recommended procedure for measuring hearing aid's, 25; assistive devices and change in, 24; as a function of input level, 25; level dependent, 20–21; selecting, 8
Frequency selectivity, 2

Gennum Corporation, 8
GN Danavox hearing aid, 8

Hawkins, D. B., 19
Hearing aid performance, recent developments in measurements of, 25–26
Hearing aid measurements, major changes in, 27
Hearing aids: bandwidth of, 4, 13–14; difficulty in adjusting to use of, 2; interfacing assistive

devices with, 24–25; major changes in, 27; with more than one type of compression, 18–19; processing in, 12–24; recent developments in, 3–4, 5, 6, 7, 8–9; tinniness in, 13. *See also names of different types and makes of hearing aids*
Hearing aid users, 1
Hearing loss: filtering technology and steeply sloping, 1; filters for flat and mildly sloping 12; filters for normal hearing in low frequency and steeply sloping high frequency, 12–13; fitting person with upward sloping, 13; individual differences in sensorineural, 2; need to identify characteristics of, 28; sensorineural, 1, 2; steeply sloping high frequency, 13
High pass filter switch, 20

Individual differences: in benefit from noise reduction hearing aid, 22; in sensorineural hearing loss, 2
Induction loops, 24
In-the-ear hearing aids, 9–10
Infrared listening systems, 24
Input-output characteristics of compression system, 14–16
Input-output function of hearing aid, 25–26
Intrason France, 8

Level-dependent frequency response, 20–21
Linear hearing aid, multiband hearing aid advantge over, 18
Loudness discomfort, 2

Microphones: directional, 19–20; electret, 13
Miniaturization, 27
Multiband adaptive filter, 22
Multiband hearing aid, 27; consistent advantage over linear hearing aid, 18